Peter Valenta

Utopian Belief and Plausibility

Sketches of an Ideal

Peter Valenta

**UTOPIAN BELIEF
AND PLAUSIBILITY**
Sketches of an Ideal

⸻

Original German Title:
Utopischer Glaube und Plausibilität
Skizzen eines Ideals

Copyright © 2022 Peter Valenta
All rights reserved.

Contact: valenta.peter@t-online.de

Cover design and graphics :Marii Brédard
Translation :Danny McPherson
Proof-reading and editing :Catriona Valenta

ISBN: 978-3-00-071679-9

For Robert
(11. 06. 1991 – 01. 07. 1991)

"Do you realise, however, how much easier devout enthusiasm is than good action?"

(Nathan the Wise[1])

Deo gratias.[2]

---

[1] Gotthold Ephraim Lessing, (1729 – 1781), German writer

[2] for all His help in the creation of this book

Content

Introduction	9
The Ideal	15
Epilogue	70
Sources	74

Introduction

Who am I to write about such a vast topic? I am a technician and businessman and have been working with technical equipment and industrial machinery for over fifty years. But I am interested in philosophical, political, social and religious developments in our society. On the one hand, I find that all that has happened in the past few decades encouraging, but I cannot close my eyes and ears to the suffering and grievances that exist on so many levels. However, as many have said before me: *hope dies last.* I still feel a sense of hope driving my heart, and surprisingly - more often than I would suspect - my brain confirms it too: the perception of positive developments. For me, the glass is usually half full.

Universal ethical values are my concern, and these should, as a matter of urgency, be further explored, as Albert Henry Halsey[3] stated: *'The beginning of the change that will enable the human species to survive is to be found precisely in the search for universal values. We need to take this much more seriously than we do at present.'*

I would like to try to work out, based on my own life experiences, what is plausible for me in matters of faith and what I can and still want to represent after all the scandals within various religious institutions. In doing so, I would like to stress that my little booklet can only provide a sketch of things that are immeasurably more complex in the dimensions of the physical and spiritual worlds. Even if some things seem

---

[3] (1923–2014), British sociologist

abbreviated or simplified, I ask you, the readers, to view my text as a prompt.

The vast majority of people, even in the most far-flung parts of the world, have access to the internet. With global news technology, which can be a blessing as well as a curse, we are kept constantly informed or misinformed. One thing is clear: through this technology, we are updated in real time - and on a local and global level - not only about the weather, but also about the conflict-ridden state of our world. It goes without saying that there is a great deal of common ground among all people on this earth, in the sense that we *all* strive for love, happiness, joy, prosperity and freedom. And so it is not surprising that rituals, religions, ideas and ideologies, good and bad, have arisen, all with noble aims and good intentions to make the world a better place. Indeed, outwardly we have come a long way, but what about our *spiritual* climate? Many are justifiably concerned about the earth's climate, but shouldn't our spiritual climate be at the top of our list of priorities?

The big final question remains: does God exist? And does this Creator - whatever we understand or have learned about Him - have a plan, a heart for us humans, regardless of our tradition or religion?

A few years ago, I heard a physicist give a lecture in Giessen. He spoke about things at the limits of our comprehension, the universe and its beginnings. A very long time ago, essentially at *zero hour,* the universe was sparked into existence, and today in the 21st century a physicist asks himself: *who* was that? *Who* made the big bang? In addition to numerous other astonishing scientific facts, he also shared a universally relatable parable:

Piano music, and where mice believe it comes from:

The mice ask themselves where the piano music comes from. They arrive at a mystical story about the existence of humans. Then they begin to investigate. They discover hammers and strings. They see this as the explanation and say: 'There are no humans. The music comes from little hammers.'

Although their conclusion is correct, it is still not enough! As the physicist pointed out-someone made the piano, someone composed and played the music.

Coming from the Roman Catholic tradition of the memorial acclamation[4], I was moved in the spring of 1978[i] by the

---

[4] Acclamation sung or recited by the congregation after the institution narrative of the Eucharist.

vision of a plausible convergence of faith, reason and science.

The text in this small booklet may seem like a "no-brainer" to some readers - things that there is no real need to discuss, let alone write about. But perhaps my text will help against the degradation of our intellectual climate and provide a little hope and confidence in these difficult times - or serve as a stimulus for the reader's own search for universal values.

Spring 2022

The Ideal

It should be possible to form a consensus based on universal principles. The physicist Max Planck once said that religion and science complement one another. There is far more than that which meets the eye.

It is probable that the fundamental questions about life and the universe can only be answered satisfactorily when we first spiritually perceive the essence and inner heart of the great mover, God.

But the invisible being for me - God - can be fathomed and understood through His creation. The sciences are approaching the invisible, the mystical and the mysterious, which means that faith can no longer be dismissed as mere 'irrationality'. The concepts of *cause* (energy) and *effect* (matter) can be plausibly applied to an artist or creator and his works. You can certainly find fitting passages on this in the Holy Scriptures. I want to make as few theological references as possible in my text, because the goal of religion should be to fade into the background as soon as we ignorant human beings are reconnected with our Creator, i.e. when we know and truly *live* a spiritual life.

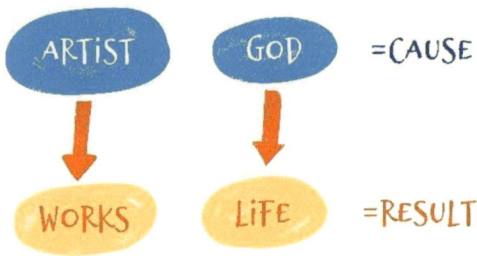

Figure 1

All things have an inner nature or character and an outer form or matter and structure. Furthermore, all things exist with polar characteristics, from particles, atoms, molecules, plants, animals - all the way up to mankind. That is, in everything there is an inherent directional nature or mind, and in man, exclusively, a compassionate consciousness capable of self-reflection. These polar characteristics also include positivity and negativity (as in particles and atoms) as well as masculine and feminine elements in plants and animals, manifested in humans as *man* and *woman,* although it is indisputable that men have some feminine aspects and women some masculine aspects. Everything serves processes of mutual complementation and development. The Asian yin-yang symbol ☯ illustrates this vividly. Then there are the concepts of *subject* and *object*. The subject and object positions are never just static or rigid; subject[5] and object are always coupled with processes, the goal of which is always the pursuit of the optimum. Everything can only exist in relationship.

Of course, I am aware that such a short description is a vast over-simplification and that everything behind these outlined words and diagrams is infinitely more complex.

But if I assume that God is the first cause of all beings from the smallest particles up to humankind, then it follows that God, as symbolically depicted in nature, should also carry the polar characteristics of being within Himself. But because God is invisible, one wonders how these polar

---

[5] Werner Heisenberg remarked in an interview in 1968 that the relationship between subject and object in atomic physics did not look as simple as it did in classical physics.

characteristics (inner-outer, positive-negative[6], male-female) can be explained in the Creator Himself? If God is the first source of being, then one might assume that without God, the universe would potentially collapse.

Even if God is not visible to us, God's *exterior* might be considered as a *universal source of energy* that works ceaselessly and keeps everything in the universe turning. At the next level, towards the core of God's being, we can recognise *laws, ideas, will, reason*, and yes - even *emotions*.

When I think of *laws*, for example, I think of the force of gravity, the centrifugal force, the intrinsic rotation of the planets and the orbiting of planets around the sun. The balance of all these forces is more than incredible.

---

[6] Not in the sense of good and evil

When I think of God's *ideas*, it is not only the ingenious functioning of my eyes and brain that come to mind; but *the capacity I have to be creative myself.*

When I think of God's *reason,* I ask myself how it is even possible that life exists here on earth at all, in such a narrow corridor of the universe. To give just two examples: the finely tuned temperature range and life-sustaining oxygen levels within the earth's atmosphere. Only a few kilometres away from earth, the environment becomes lethal for us.

Concerning God's *will,* historians tell us that human history shows a positive trend towards freedom, religious understanding and world peace. People living under totalitarian regimes are fighting back and the number of dictatorships decreasing.

How can we interpret God's *emotions?* Consider how the beautiful shapes, colours and scents of a flower appeal to our emotions, and how gracefully, gently and vibrantly a beautiful butterfly flutters before our eyes in the summer sunlight.

Can I simply assign all these qualities to God, or are we human beings in fact the *essential image* of the first, enduring Creator? And are these objects the *symbolic image* of the first great Mover? But what is the innermost core of the Creator? Does God have a *heart* (in the sense of a centre emotion, intellect and morality), and if so, what qualities are contained within?

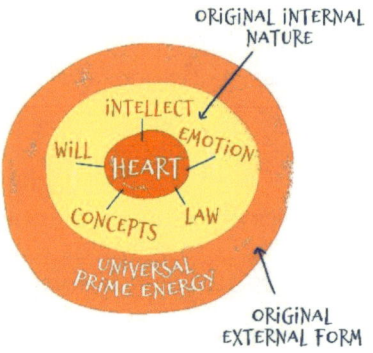

Figure 2

Based on these bold assumptions, I reflect on the relationship between God and all creation. Assuming there is a reason for creation, this invisible cause, regardless of whether I can imagine it or not, created a visible object and nothing can come from nothing. What then is man's role vis-à-vis God? Do we have free will, and why? Did the Creator assign a co-creator role to the mature human being? In Figure 3, God's relationship with all creation is outlined in a very simplified way.

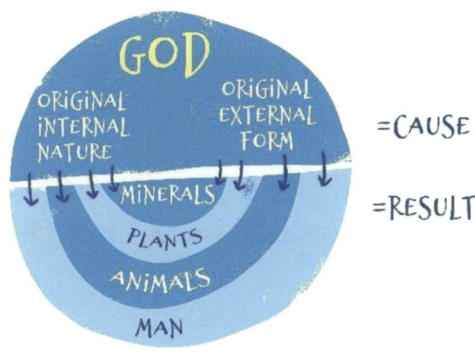

Figure 3

No creature exists independently of another, but rather it is made and formed in such a way to bring life and benefit to others through mutual relationships; think of the interaction between flower, bee and honey. Healthy and optimal reciprocal relationships produce all the forces required for existence, reproduction, maintenance and action, all fed by a universal original energy.

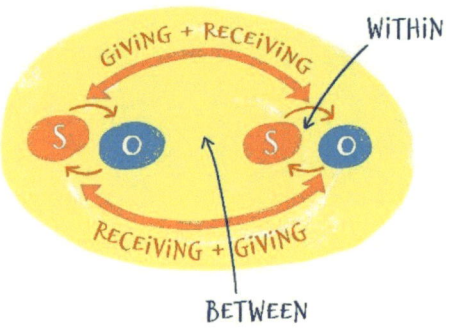

Figure 4

This principle of *give* and *receive* runs through the entire structure of the universe, right down to the physical body of man including his spirit and interpersonal relationships. Many examples could be listed here. The same principle applies from the smallest on earth to the "ultra-deep field[7]"; from cation (plus) and anion (minus) to the interactions between suns and planets. There are horizontal and vertical forces of give and receive. With vertical, we may think of God's constant universal energy source and with horizontal, its flow between and within his creations. I find it logical that in the universe, which we can perceive and estimate with our eyes, there are invisible fields of force (e.g. magnetism and others such as radiation) which have been observable since time immemorial and are now being increasingly and more precisely investigated by scientific consensus.

---

[7] Hubble Telescope (HUDF)

The universe was not created by God in the biblical literal six days, but, as scientific evidence shows, in successive, prolonged phases of time. All created beings go through processes of growth[8] that require time. Examples from nature illustrate this, such as the three stages of most plants (root, stem, flower).

At some point in life, we all ask ourselves: why do I exist? And what motivated mankind to invent such incredible and complex things in our short time of existence, while we have remained relatively backward in our relationships with one another? Does the Creator not care? And if not, what would the relationship between God and man look if it were to have a positive impact on the world? Something[9] all too often inhibits

---

[8] Formation. growth, completion

[9] In religious terms, *the Fall of Man*

good relationships between people. At this point I would like to address the concept of *perfection*. By this, I am not referring to *perfectionism*. The perfection of an enchanting rose delights my mind, even if one of its petals is not without flaw - it is nevertheless unique and enchants my senses with its fragrance, its luminous colour and its *perfect,* flawless form and appearance. When applied to humans, however, the concept of *perfection* produces unease and stress in me, as the bar is set so very high. What is more, terrible tyrants the world over have unashamedly exploited and abused our human longing for ideal conditions. That is why I prefer to use the term *mature* character, meaning *inner* and *outer* maturity. Should the Creator have intended something far more noble with us humans than with a rose? Does God want us humans to reflect His *perfection* and love? More than that - are we even ideally the reciprocal and potential partner of the Creator?

The universe appears to be self-sufficient. Long before life came into being and became possible on earth, there were already countless galaxies, and the universe is still expanding, even now. I seriously ask myself: if God exists, does this divinity want to be in a love relationship with us humans, a mutual, loving relationship? What might this relationship look like, beyond religion, sacrifices, rituals and prayers?

The concepts of *heart* and *motive* are key concepts in the understanding of the origin of humans and our relationship with God. If God, like *ideal parents,* has a loving inner heart that beats for His essential image - the human being - as well as His symbolic creation, then this assumption raises further profound thoughts and questions: *is there in God an emotional state such as longing?* In what way would God have prepared us so that we could continually experience this connection? A *natural divine spirituality*[10] would be required. How would such a society look and function? External approaches to this are already being discussed and experimented with, for example the 'economy for the common good.' But what would such a society look like in interpersonal terms?[11]

I would like to understand even more deeply and ask: how does something new come into being? I cannot answer this scientifically, but I can cite a few observations from nature. In all living beings there is a force that values the *purpose of the whole* more highly than the *purpose of the self*. In the *origin* - the

---

[10] Not religiosity or esotericism

[11] Book tip: Moral 4.0 by Hubert Thurnhofer

Creator - subject and object aspects must also exist, otherwise *subjects* and *objects* could not combine in matter in such a special way as *one,* and form a new unit or union, a synthesis.

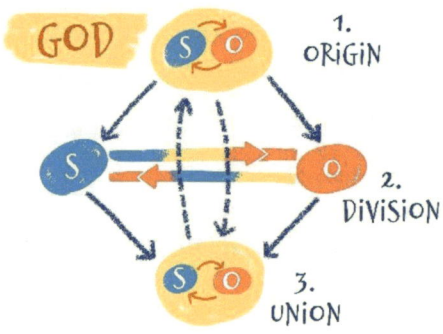

Figure 5

This synthesis, a new object, has the amazing potential to become a subject itself. Is it not incredible that the positions of the subject and object can vary and are dynamic and not rigid?

Within these *four positions,* six different basic relationships of give and receive are possible. For *subject* we can insert *spirit* of a human being and for *object* the human *body* and the resulting *union* is a *mature human being.* This example makes it clear that the subject and object roles are not static. My mind as subject can *discipline* my body as object telling it to exercise and eat moderately, and similarly, my exhausted or sick body can be subject and demand, even force, recovery and rest - even against my will. This pattern can be applied universally to family, society and the relationship between man and the natural world.

The purpose of creation is to experience joy and love and is at the core of all existence. Everything has a purpose for its existence conceived by its Creator. If a product loses its reason for being, it should be repaired, recycled or reused. Awareness of a preserving *cradle-to-cradle* philosophy which preserves, rather than a *cradle-to-grave* philosophy, is increasing. This means that in the conception process (logos), consideration is given to what use an item can have after its life cycle and how materials can be recycled and conserved in the most environmentally friendly way possible. With these considerations, money and profit will not be determining factors in the future. If items such as satellites, cars, and electrical appliances already have such an important purpose, how much more important is the purpose of a human being?

A created object does not decide its own purpose; that is determined by its creator or designer. Therefore, it would be beneficial to know quite impartially and free from any ideology, the intention of the Creator with His creation, so that I can logically and plausibly understand the purpose of my existence as well as that of the cosmos around me and thus act accordingly for the benefit of all.

What moved the Almighty, the Eternal, the Absolute, to create? The concepts of *motive* and *heart* are connected. Heart is the urge to love an object and the hope for reciprocation. If God's essential aspect is His heart, then heart is also the essence of our personality and character. The heart has the impulse to love and to be completely united in love with the object of its love, whereby, ideally, even the roles of subject and object become irrelevant, because such unity - mentally or spiritually - takes on spherical, circular forms. The heart then becomes the source of love from which all motivation for action springs for the benefit of the object and subject partner (for example, man *and* woman). Such a unity would be inseparable and resistant to any disturbing impulses.

It is God's love or heart that seeks the most diverse forms of expression. It is in the nature of the heart to seek an object that it can love. This is how creation comes into being and how it finds its fulfilment. It is the source and inspiration of love.

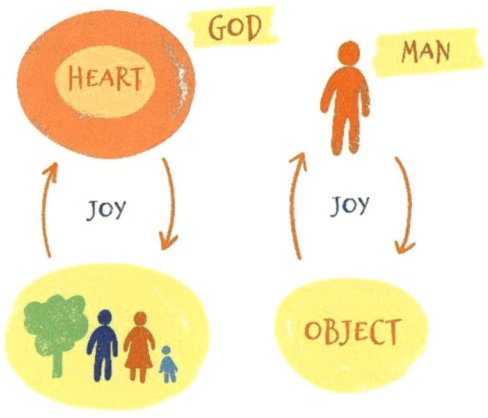

Figure 6

If the Creator possesses such a heart and the creation arose from God's Logos, then this means that God, whose innermost essence is heart, feels joy when He can love an object that He has created. If there is no object, God cannot satisfy His urge to express care, compassion and love. God made creation as an object that He could love.

When I think about how joy comes about, or how I feel joy, I quickly realise, especially in times of the pandemic-imposed quarantine and curfews, that joy does not usually come from a single person alone. We need friends or an object in which, at least in some respects, our own being can be reflected. A painter is happy when he or she has a vision or idea of a stimulating object, and is even more happy when the idea appears in front of him or her as a successful painting which then also brings joy to a loved one. We are most excited by relationships with people, animals, nature or material objects. Surely this quality in man must come from the Creator. From this I can deduce that God must be pleased when His original being is physically, and spiritually reflected in His creation. Therefore, *man,* rather than angels, as understood by some religions, has the potential to be closest to the heart of God as a reciprocating being.

The development of a living being is subject to a process of growth or maturation, which can be roughly divided into three stages: formation, growth and completion. The growth process needs special protection. For example, in nature, a sudden onset of wintry conditions in early spring can disrupt or even destroy the first tender shoots of a vine. But these are merely external disruptive elements. Psychological problems can arise during human development. Almost all cultures and religions describe a major original event when mankind was separated from the Creator. The biblical story told in my culture is that God's act of creation had a successful beginning but was followed by the expulsion of the first human beings from paradise because they disobeyed a commandment. How can we return there?

I can try to explain this from my own experience. My first profession (1970-1974) was a radio and television mechanic and my whole professional life has consisted of fixing things. In order to be able to fix a malfunctioning radio, I need first to have some understanding of the concept, the plan and the purpose, i.e. the ideal state of the radio. Only then is it possible to effectively diagnose the problem and carry out a successful repair. It is always an uplifting and good feeling for me when something works again, but it gives me even more pleasure when I see the eyes of the customer light up as an old, but still usable device or industrial machine fulfils its purpose once again. Compared to a technical device, no matter how intricate, the human mind and psyche is incomparably more complex and interwoven with countless dynamic networks.

If I assume that our Creator, out of a motive of the heart, assigned an intelligent and loving purpose to us human beings, then we could speak of three related tasks each of which has an individual and the higher purpose of loving horizontal interpersonal relationships and the vertical, equally loving mutual relationship between God and mankind. The Bible[12] uses the

---

[12] Genesis 1:28

term *blessing* to describe these three tasks. Is this possibly the Creator's unequivocal core message for our existence? This short passage right at the beginning of the Bible is, after all, the consensus found across the three Abrahamic[13] world religions. The four-position diagram (Fig. 5) is the basis on which God functions. As we take responsibility and grow through fulfilling the great blessings, we fulfil the divine ideal of love on earth and brings perfect joy to God and man.

If these fundamentals had been realised, we would have inherited God's character and made God's nature our own, and God would always be naturally, without prayers and sacrifices, at the centre of our thoughts, feelings and actions. There would be no

---

[13] Judaism, Christianity and Islam

competition between religions or ideologies.

The first blessing *(be fruitful* means to become physically and spiritually mature).

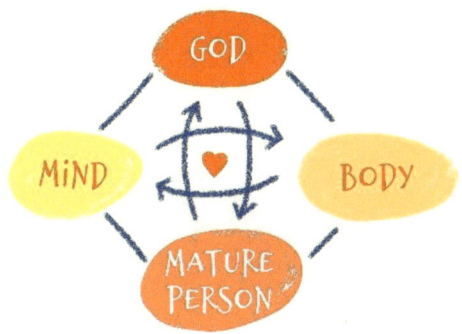

Figure 7

Such a person could not possibly commit a crime, for he would himself feel the same suffering that he would thereby inflict on God, his Creator. A human being would be the fruit of God's vertical love and would feel this connection as immediate and personal. Nowadays there are many ways to develop an individual and unique personality.

Who do I want to be? ....

The second blessing (*multiply and replenish the earth* means to create an exclusive man-woman relationship, have a family and then extend to family, society, nation and the world).

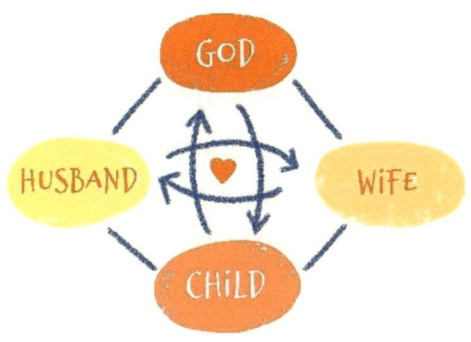

Figure 8

The second task or blessing is, as a mature individual, to establish a family and procreate new life. God's vertical love expresses itself in parental love on earth.

God surely intended that man should realise His love horizontally and have children and, in this way, experience himself God's creativity. From the perspective of the heart, this is a great blessing and joy, because only through having children of one's own[14] can man completely and uniquely experience the vertical love of God and fully understand how God feels towards man. The spirit and heart of strong families shapes society and radiates out into the world.

---

[14] Not necessarily one's biological child but also a foster child, adopted child, or godchild.

The third blessing (*subdue and have dominion over the fish of the sea, and over the fowl of the air, and over every living thing that moveth upon the earth*).

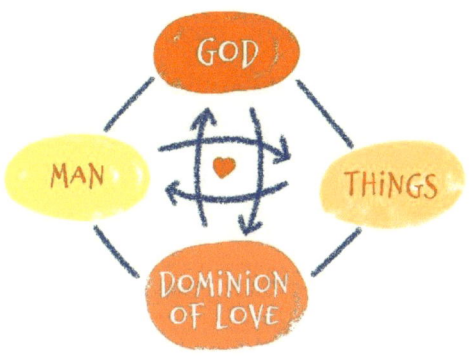

Figure 9

The third blessing makes it clear that the Creator gave man the right to care for the whole of creation and the earth's atmosphere in a prudent, intelligent and loving way. The awkwardly formulated term 'dominion' can be better understood by ideas of sustainability, such as the previously mentioned *cradle-to-cradle* philosophy. Man can lovingly and responsibly take care of the earth as the Creator would, and in doing so feel deep, satisfying joy and gratitude for himself and for the world.

Before God created man, He created all things in the image (concept) of man. Therefore, the external structures, functions and characteristics found in the animal world are the same as those found in man. Similarly, we find the characteristics of plants and minerals in man. This could mean that, even before the Creator began creating, the motive of his love[15] for man took a central role, and God thus intended there to be an exceptional, special position for humankind. The world in which *the three great blessings* are realised would therefore be the ideal world, in which God and man, as well as man and the cosmos, are in balance and harmony. Such a world would certainly be the Kingdom of Heaven on earth.

The three blessings described earlier exist simultaneously. They are highly dynamic and intertwined and exist unselfishly for the benefit of all. As already mentioned, today's world has become enormously complicated. However, the best possible world in the future will also be very complex, but without the current aspects of self-interest. It could be said that the

---

[15] Only possible with freedom, responsibility, maturity etc.

Kingdom of Heaven is like a human being who has attained *maturity of character* (perfection). There would be no conflict between physical and spiritual desires.

In humans, the impulses of the physical mind are transmitted to the entire body via the central nervous system and stimulate actions that serve its self-preservation. Likewise, no healthy part of the body will ever rebel against the impulses of the healthy nervous system, just as the mature human being would not rebel against God's *dominion of love* (parenthood). In such a world there would be no destructive strife and no crime. Nevertheless, it would not be boring because our stricken spiritual senses would be restored and open to the wonderful things that at present, at best, only flicker magically in isolated instances. People would live for each other in a way not imaginable at the present time and would naturally make their contribution to family, society and nation. The purpose of the whole (solidarity-community) has a secondary aim of improvement of the individual. The purpose of the self, therefore, does not stand separately and competitively in the way of the purpose of the whole. The purpose of the whole could not continue to exist without guaranteeing an end in itself. The whole of creation is an organic body that is woven and interconnected by highly complex, polar, reciprocal purposes - there is far more than we can see. With this consciousness, we would be able to find solutions to problems much more effectively and quickly. Giving joy selflessly thus simultaneously guarantees that human beings can experience the greatest possible joy in all relationships as well as shared trust. We would deal with our mistakes much more lovingly and constructively.

How does God connect with His creations, especially with man - directly, and/or in-directly? It can be assumed that after successfully passing through the three stages of growth, a direct connection between man and his Creator would be possible. There would be no need for religions, prayers and sacrifices. Love and truth as well as intelligent processes for optimisation would always have universal joy and happiness in view. We would be permanently in a special sphere of direct divine connection and would, with curiosity and in a very natural way, be able to recognise God's heart and being, like pieces of a puzzle, in every fellow human being. The Creator would govern all things indirectly through man. Such a trust of God towards us earth-dwellers is to be embraced with true love.

The fact that our earth is not doing well has nothing to do with plants, insects and animals, but with unwise, immature, and poorly thought-out decisions made by humans.

Now the question is, how does God *govern* (guide) man while he is still in the process of growth - that is, still *immature*? At this point, the commandments of God in the Bible play a role. It should be clear that a growing child needs certain restrictions or rules for protection. Most of the rules become superfluous once the child reaches a more mature state. Loving parents do not issue rules on a whim or because they want to test their children, but rather out of love and for their own protection. My image of God is that of a loving God whose love for his creation corresponds to the heart of mature parents who have only the very best in mind for their beloved children. God's commandment was only necessary during man's growth phase. God took such an enormously high risk with man because of the nature of His love towards us. True love is only possible in complete freedom, and here individual responsibility and the ability to make decisions play an important role. Nature has no choice; a tree grows and thrives according to its inherent directional nature. Nature is *only*[16] the symbolic image of God, which cannot respond directly to its Creator. We humans are longed for and desired by God on an astonishingly high level, equipped with the ability to surprise even the Creator. That is why God gave us our own share of responsibility. We were to qualify as lord (and lady) over the cosmos. The actual right to direct dominion belongs

---

[16] "Only" - with respect and humility in the face of nature

only to the Creator. Nevertheless, God wanted man to be able to rule all things. In order for man to rightfully and correctly exercise this positive dominion, the Creator had to implant or bequeath to us the essence of His ability to create. For this purpose, man should voluntarily participate in his own process of creation and thus gratefully and appreciatively accept God's inheritance. Unlike animals and plants, human beings do not develop to maturity through principles and energy alone. Our exclusive, necessary contribution to this is *our* own responsibility, which is very small in comparison to God's.

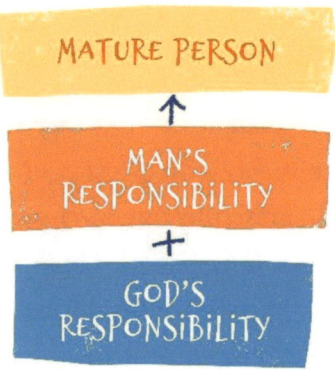

Graphic 10

The Creator cannot intervene in man's personal sphere of responsibility, for that would mean that God is fallible and would violate His own high principle of love. God must have taken such an enormously high risk *only* to begin a true love relationship with us humans.

Our freedom and responsibility to handle love properly is a precious grace that God grants us. If this is true, then it is not wise to place any blame on the Creator for any unsolved problems on earth; even asking why God allows evil to happen is rather misplaced.

The world consists not only of the *visible physical* world, which one could compare with the human body, but also of an *invisible substantial world*.

We can better understand the relationship between these two worlds by looking at the relationship between mind and body. Our physical body is limited by time; it does not go beyond the present moment. It is a *being of the moment* and with time it ages and returns to dust. Our mind is not limited by time; if it wants to, it can freely think about the past and imagine the future. It is eternal. The physical body is also limited by space and cannot be in more than one place at a time. The mind, on the other hand, is not limited by space. It leaves no visible traces in the spatial world and can, if it wishes, dwell in any place. The mind is so infinite that it can encompass the universe when it expands. The sphere of action of the limited, transient body is the visible physical world, while the unlimited, eternal mind lives in the invisible but substantial world. Just as the human mind is the subject, impulse and sense-giver of the body, so the invisible world is the subject, impulse and sense-giver of the visible world. Both worlds are inseparably united in the living human being.

What is the relationship of the human being to these two worlds? The *physical self* of the human being consists of the basic elements of the visible physical world. The spirit of man, the *spiritual self*, was created from the elements of the spiritual world (logos). The position of man in the cosmos is that of the microcosm in the macrocosm. God created the universe *before*[17] man, according to the pattern and structures of the dual characteristics of beings, whereupon He *later*[18] intended to create the ideal man. Man's *spiritual self* encloses the invisible substantial world within itself like a transparent bubble, while his *physical self* proverbially *grasps* the visible world.

In conclusion, it is logical for me to assume that God intended to create man as lord (and lady) of both cosmic worlds. This

---

[17] Genesis 1, 1-26
[18] Genesis 1, 27

is evident, among other things, in our quest to explore space, the moon and the fourth planet[19] of our relatively small solar system.

Man has five physical senses as well as five spiritual senses. As a result of the initial separation from the Creator, or biblical Fall of Man, our spiritual senses were impaired, and humans partially lost the ability to perceive the spiritual world. People whose spiritual senses have been restored can perceive the spiritual world quite naturally, without drugs. We live in an *evil*[20] and at the same time a *relatively good* world and the fact that we can only perceive the spiritual world to a limited extent may even be a form of protection. People who are not healthy in their soul or mind, who possibly hear voices giving instructions which are a threat to their own life or that of another,

---

[19] Mars

[20] Not in the sense of black & white thinking

or who are unable to cope well with their daily life should definitely seek professional help. Such phenomena have little to do with the outlined ideal and connection with God.

In order to get through times of difficulty, it is important to create good conditions, maintaining a mentally and physically healthy lifestyle by not taking any kind of mind-altering drugs and practising prayer or meditation[21] and exercising as well as maintaining good friend-ships.

God clearly intended man to be the mediator between the two worlds - the centre of balance and harmony in the whole creation. Man has never been able to fully assume and fulfil this honourable position in a way worthy of his Creator. The

---

[21] In balance, without overdoing it!

painting[22] on the next page perfectly illustrates the meaning of this quotation from the Bible.

We know that the whole creation has been groaning and travailing in pain until now.

Romans 8:22

---

[22] Johannes Seewald - 1982

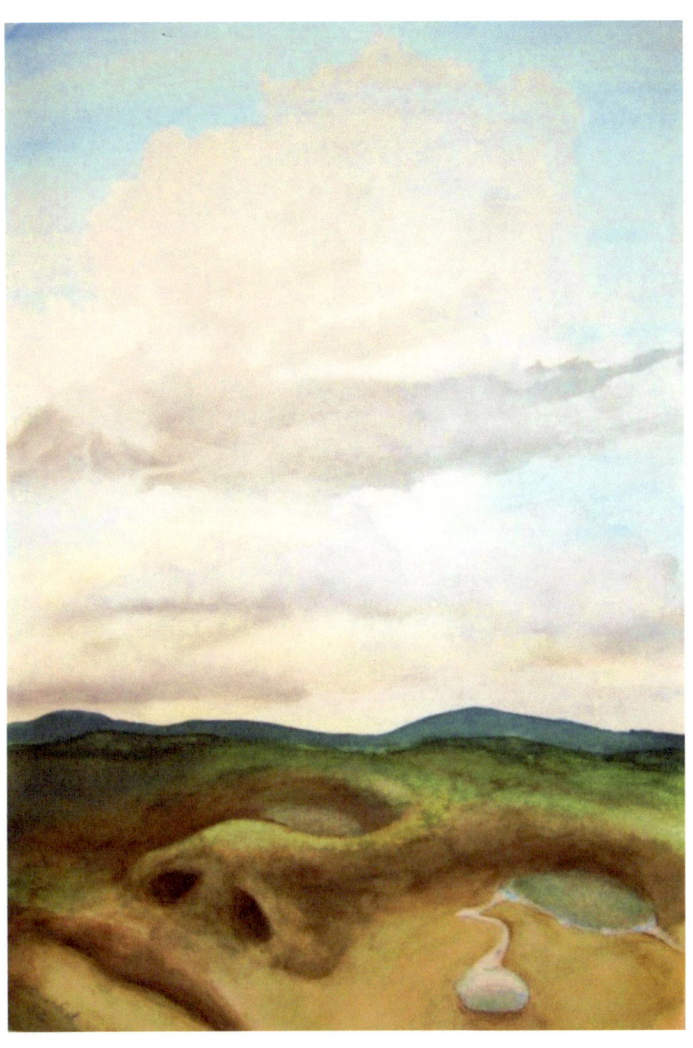

In order to be able to grow in a healthy way, the *physical self* needs air and sunlight as well as water and a wide variety of foodstuffs. The *spiritual self* also needs nourishment for its growth and maturity. Ideally, it receives life elements - love and truth -from parents who represent God. In this way the human heart and mind can develop and mature in truth and love. If the *physical self* acts in accordance with God's purpose, it transmits positive elements of vitality to encourage growth of the *spiritual self*. However, the *spiritual self* not only *receives*, but also *gives* a certain element - the spirit element - back to the *physical self*. One could call these spirit elements a natural drug. This element gives joy to the *physical self* and gives energy and strength to the body.

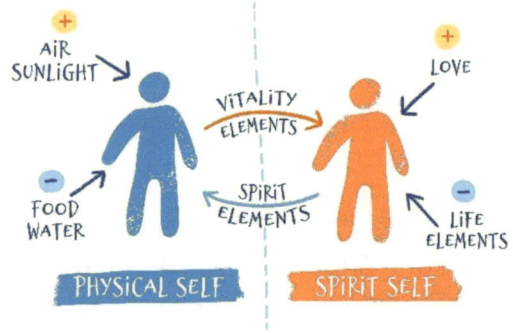

Figure 11

The quality or level of the *spiritual self* thus also depends on the physical actions performed by an individual. Bad actions can damage or 'kill' the *spiritual self*, which may be even more tragic than the death of the physical body. Good physical actions, on the other hand, transfer positive vitality elements to the *spiritual self*. A person with an *evil* [23]*spiritual self* who wants to change and become good, must repent, ideally while still on earth. The *evil spiritual self* can become whole if it receives elements of vitality through true repentance, faith in God and good actions[24]. Faith in God alone is not enough. This principle works universally, even if a person does not believe in God. The perception of God's love has much to do with how we are raised. Striving to establish a good relationship between the *spiritual* and *physical self* enables one to come closer to God and will have positive effects. If a person strives for this and lives in balance according to his own conscience, the Kingdom of Heaven will already begin in his heart. The world into which his refined *spiritual self* enters after his life on earth will be the Kingdom

---

[23] Evil is relative

[24] Repairing damage, making amends, at least symbolically.

of Heaven in the spiritual world. Because life in the visible real world plays such a decisive role, Jesus taught the great wisdom[25]:

> ...Whatsoever ye shall bind on earth shall be bound in heaven; and whatsoever ye shall loose on earth shall be loosed in heaven...
> Matthew 18:18

The truth of these words of Jesus is often seen in people who are slowly and consciously coming to the end of their life. Things come to light that would never have been thought possible. For example, a dying person who has seemingly led an irreproachable private and public life and had a faithful and exemplary marriage, may admit to an adultery that had been kept secret for a long time.

---

[25] Matthew 18:18

It seems obvious to me that it is not God who decides on the judgement day whether or not a person will go to heaven, but that each person decides this himself through his daily life on earth.

In summary, I understand that our original spirit, breathed into us by God, strives towards a give and take between our *physical* and our *spiritual self*, which is oriented towards the original reference point of our Creator - absolute true love.

In a future world, one that may appear utopian from today's point of view, there will still be old age, disease and death. But our ability to maintain conditions for the success of life, love and happiness will be far greater than it is at the present time. That is my vision.

My conscience is my ethical compass which guides me towards good thoughts and actions. It is a valuable and fragile instrument, a gauge to be used every day on our journey through this meaningful, exciting and beautiful life on our unique planet Earth. Ideally, physical death is not a funeral service, but a redemptive celebration of joy after a fulfilling life. Similar to the birth of a much desired and beloved child but a new life begins in another dimension.

The butterfly often forgets
that it was once a caterpillar.

From Sweden

Epilogue

I have asked many questions and tried to highlight what still resonates in my naïve, childlike heart, even though it all may seem unrealistic, and I am about to turn sixty-seven. It is my dream, my hope for the utopia of a better world that gives me unwavering courage.

I am including an incomplete list of the books that I have been reading lately:

- The Book That Made Your World – Vishal Mangalwadi
- The Old Man and the Sea – Ernest Hemingway
- Aus, Amen, Ende? – Thomas Frings
- When Nietzsche Wept – Irvin D. Yalom
- Der eigen-sinnige Mensch – Helmut Milz

- Realizing Jesus – Kevin McCarthy
- Schuldig – Thomas Middelhof
- Moral 4.0 – Hubert Thurnhofer
- Nathan und seine Kinder – Mirjam Pressler
- The Courage To Be – Paul Tillich
- The Good Book of Human Nature– Carel van Schaik and Kai Michel
- Farewell Sidonia – Erich Hackl
- Barracoon – Zora Neale Hurston
- An Appeal by the Dalai Lama to the World: Ethics are More Important than Religion – Franz Alt
- Gott befreit von Religion – Florian Kliman
- Das Buch der Freude – Dalai Lama and Tutu
- Die kleinste gemeinsame Wirklichkeit – Mai Thi Nguyen-Kim
- Zeitenwende 1979 – Frank Bösch

- Iron John – Robert Bly

I think that we are living in a time in which ideological and religious disputes are no longer of primary importance. Instead, what matters is interdenominational understanding, the questioning and searching for possibilities which can allow the different traditions and cultures to live together based on common ethical values. This requires efforts that go far beyond religious ideas.

Just as there is an international system of units for physical constants, so should an internationally recognised system of units for spiritual, ethical values be developed and bindingly adopted by all states and their related organisations. The only existing equivalent is the United Nations' Universal Declaration of Human Rights. I realise that this is a huge task, and many different voices want to make themselves heard. Interreligious dialogues are already happening. Such an ethical *gold standard,* once ratified by all states, should be unlimited in time and non-negotiable.

Is this the utopian demand of a naïve man, or is it realistic, as the British sociologist Halsey urged last century? Every practicable contribution in this direction - for the good of all - is valuable and should be encouraged and appreciated.

Sources

The diagrams and much of the intellectual content of this book are, with permission of Kando Publishing, adapted from the study guide "The Principle in Outline Level 4", 1981, 1st edition, ISBN 3-922947-02-6.

The Ideal is in thyself;
the impediment too.

Thomas Carlyle (1795 – 1881)
Scottish Philosopher.

[i] In the spring of 1978, in Austria, I became acquainted with the ideas of the Unification Church. The basic principles of this teaching provide a coherent and plausible explanation of how God, spirituality, reason and science need not contradict each other. The initial contact came about through a work colleague in a machine factory. This all-important encounter has had a profound and defining influence on me to this day. Forty years after this key turning point in my life, I managed to look back in a reflective, conciliatory and self-forgiving way, and I was very grateful to be able to publish my autobiography ("Courage to be myself", ISBN 978-3-00-063291-4) in June 2019. It was an extremely important process for me to better understand why I took this path, away from the mainstream, but still in touch with society and grounded in my decades of work in industry; perhaps even why I had to take it.